SMOOTHIES
FOR WEIGHT LOSS

OVER 45 HEALTHY
GREEN SMOOTHIE RECIPES
TO DETOXIFY YOUR BODY AND
FAT BURNING DURING SIRTFOOD DIET
PHASE 1 AND 2

Dotty Branch

2

Contents

INTRODUCTION

Most people eat unhealthily in these days. Too much meat, too much fats and too much sugar are eaten. There are also a lot of ready-made meals that are full of preservatives. In the long term, this has devastating effects on health and often leads to the well-known diseases of civilization such as diabetes, cardiovascular diseases and high blood pressure, to name just a few.

Too many proteins, fats and carbohydrates are simply taken in with food, and too few vital substances such as vitamins and minerals. These valuable nutrients are mainly found in foods of plant origin, i.e. in vegetables, fruits, seeds and nuts. Especially in this day and age, when we are exposed to severe environmental pollution and a lot of stress, a healthy diet is more important than ever.

And green smoothies in particular can make a significant contribution to this. They are real powerhouses that provide energy, strengthen the immune system and help to support the internal organs (liver, kidneys, etc.) in their important functions.

In this recipe book, you will learn what green smoothies are, what ingredients the individual fruits and vegetables contain and what effect they have on your organism. You will also find tips on buying the right blender and a seasonal calendar that shows you which types of fruit and vegetables you can buy fresh from the harvest.

The recipes are divided into two main categories:

* recipes with water and recipes
* with other liquids like almond milk, coconut water or milk, apple juice and so on.

Each recipe makes 1 to 2 servings.

3 Smoothies a Day are 1000 calories.

Do not forget, you will need a good mixer to prepare all the mouth-watering smoothies.

The consistency of a smoothie is very individual and depends on your own taste. It is therefore advisable not to put too much liquid into the blender immediately. A smoothie that is too firm can easily be made more liquid, the other way round it is more complicated.
Try to use ripe fruit as much as possible. It is sweeter than unripe and therefore better suited to compensate for the slightly bitter taste of green vegetables. In addition, unripe fruit is also harder to digest.

The 46 selected recipes will make it easy for you to incorporate green smoothies into your everyday life.

Chapter 1

SIRTFOOD DETOX
GREEN SMOOTHIES

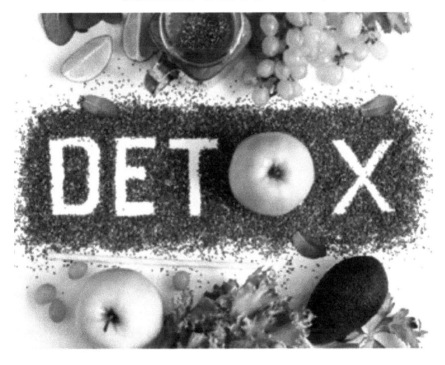

The main ingredients of green smoothies are vegetables (mostly leafy green vegetables), fruits and water or another liquid. You can add vegetal greens as well as wild herbs, seeds, nuts or other ingredients as you like.

As far as the composition is concerned, a ratio of around 60% vegetables to around 40% fruit would ideally be best. Since you have to get used to the bitter taste of green vegetables at the beginning, you can start with exactly the opposite ratio. In this book, you will find recipes with a high proportion of vegetables as well as those where the proportion of fruit predominates. After an initial phase of getting used to it, you should usemainly recipes with a high proportion of vegetables. Fruit contains a lot of fructose and therefore consuming large amounts is not recommended.

Green smoothies contain an abundance of vitamins, minerals, secondary plant substances and trace elements.

Another advantage is that chopping the ingredients releases more nutrients than would be possible by simply chewing them. In this way, our organism simply absorbs more nutrients.

The World Health Organization recommends eating 5 servings of fruit and vegetables daily. With one green smoothie a day, you'll have a large part of it covered.

Benefits of Green Smoothies

The consumption of these mixed drinks generally leads to better digestion. The whole digestive system begins to work better and more efficiently, which means that food is digested faster and better.

Because our detoxification organs (liver, gall bladder, kidneys, intestines) also work better, the toxins that we ingest through food are excreted better and faster. This not only leads to a better general sense of wellbeing, but also to a strengthening of the immune system.

Other effects of the green smoothies cannot be ignored either. The bowel movement improves, the cholesterol level is lowered and the formation of kidney and gallstones is counteracted. All of this leads to a long-term detoxification of the body and a permanent better state of health.

The green mixed drinks can also be used excellently in a weight loss diet.

It is sufficient to replace a main meal with a green smoothie. In this case, preference should be given to recipes in which the proportion of vegetables is particularly high and where only water is used, as this, unlike all other liquids, has zero calories.

Green smoothies are also particularly suitable for a detox treatment. Poor nutrition and excessive stress put a lot of strain on our internal organs and their function of eliminating toxins from our body is weakened, which can lead to various diseases. With a detoxification cure based on green smoothies, the cleansing organs (liver, kidneys, etc.) are supported in their work, which leads to an increased excretion of toxins from our organism.

Green Smoothies are also part of the Sirtfood diet. They are essential in the first part of the diet to detoxify and cleanse the body, and then in the second phase of this specific diet.

Specifically, in order to achieve the best results from the Sirtfood diet, these three phases must be followed in detail:

- Phase 1: The sirtuin diet stipulates that you should not consume more than 1,000 calories per day for the first three days. Three green juices and a solid main meal consisting of some of the foods on the sirtfood list work best. Many sirt food recipes have already been developed precisely for this phase.

- Phase 2: In the second phase, 1,500 calories are provided per day. Here you can best have two solid main meals and two juices. To slowly get your body used to foods that are not on the sirtfood list, you can add small amounts of other ingredients to your meals. This phase is carried out until the desired weight is reached.
- Phase 3: The third and final phase of the Sirt Diet is considered a sustainable change in diet. Here 1,800 calories are absorbed through food every day. Make sure, however, that you don't revert to old eating habits. The adequate intake of proteins should not be neglected either. Here it is advisable to stick to the sirtfood recipes at the beginning.

These natural smoothie recipes will also be useful for expanding your choice of juices during the first phase of the Sirtfood diet or just if you want to do a period of body cleanse.

Chapter 2

FRUIT & VEGETABLE SMOOTHIES WITH WATER

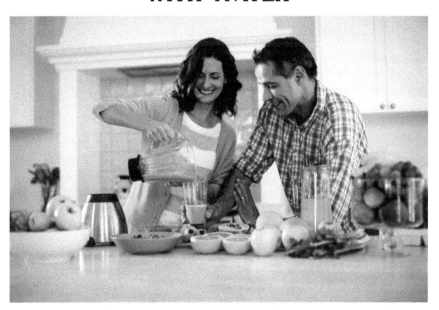

01_Spinach with Banana and Papaya

Prep time: 5 minutes
Servings: 1-2

INGREDIENTS:

- **150** G SPINACH LEAVES
- **1** SMALL BANANA
- **1/2** PAPAYA

- **100-150** ML OF WATER

DIRECTIONS:

1. Wash the vegetables, chop them roughly and put them in the blender first.

2. Then wash the fruit, remove the pits, chop and place in the blender along with any other ingredients. The peel should only be removed from types of fruit that are inedible.

3. Now add some water and mix for about 15 seconds.

4. At the end add the rest of the water until the desired consistency is achieved and mix for another 5-10 seconds.

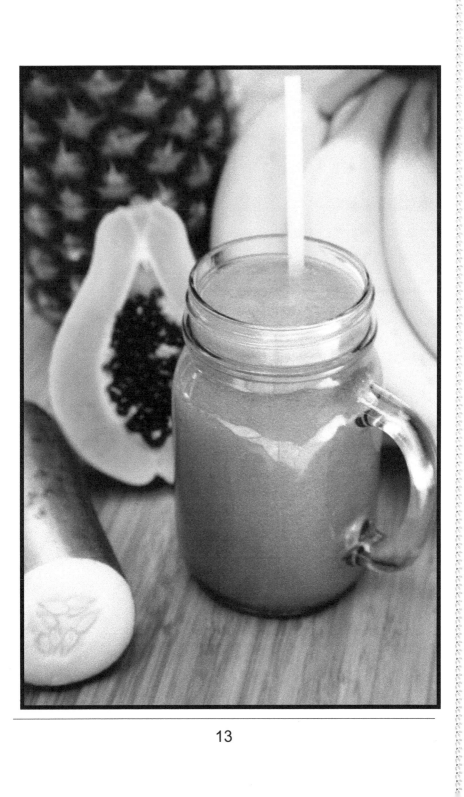

02_Spinach Chard and Kiwi

Prep time: 5 minutes
Servings: 1-2

INGREDIENTS:

- **1** HANDFUL OF SPINACH
- **2** LEAVES OF SWISS CHARD
- **1** KIWI
- **2** HANDFULS OF GRAPES

- **350**ML WATER

DIRECTIONS:

1. Wash the vegetables, chop them roughly and put them in the blender first.

2. Then wash the fruit, remove the pits, chop and place in the blender along with any other ingredients. The peel should only be removed from types of fruit that are inedible.

3. Now add some water and mix for about 15 seconds.

4. At the end add the rest of the water until the desired consistency is achieved and mix for another 5-10 seconds.

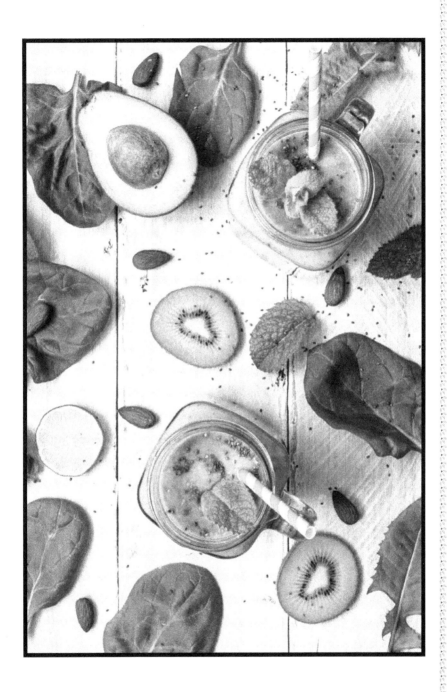

03_Spinach, Plum and Beetroot

Prep time: 5 minutes
Servings: 1-2

INGREDIENTS:

- **200** G SPINACH
- **3** PLUMS
- **100** G BEETROOT

- **200-250** ML OF WATER

DIRECTIONS:

1. Wash the vegetables, chop them roughly and put them in the blender first.

2. Then wash the fruit[1], remove the pits, chop and place in the blender along with any other ingredients. The peel should only be removed from types of fruit that are inedible.

3. Now add some water and mix for about 15 seconds.

4. At the end add the rest of the water until the desired consistency is achieved and mix for another 5-10 seconds.

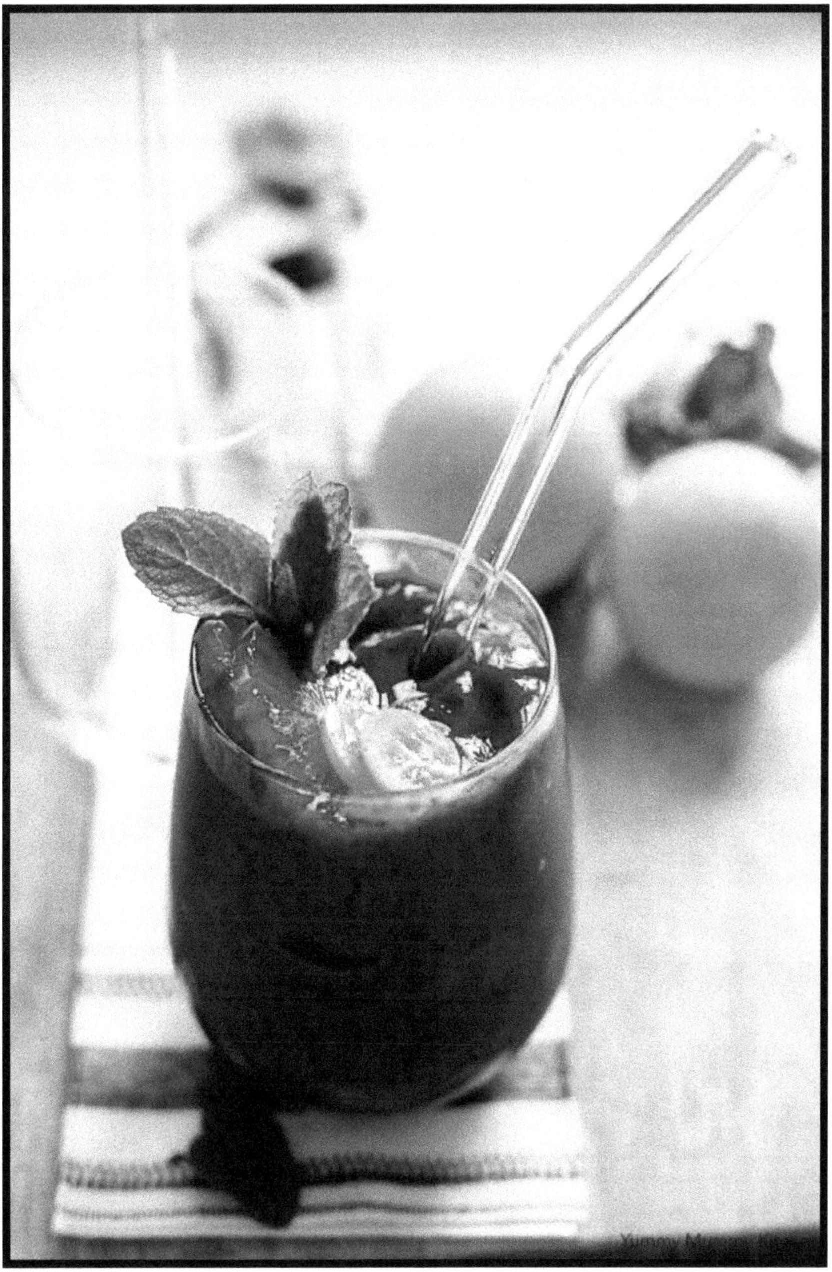

04_Spinach with Pear and Avocado

Prep time: 5 minutes
Servings: 1-2

INGREDIENTS:

- **150** G SPINACH LEAVES
- **1** MEDIUM PEAR

- **1/4** AVOCADO
- **250-300** ML OF WATER

DIRECTIONS:

1. Wash the vegetables, chop them roughly and put them in the blender first.

2. Then wash the fruit, remove the pits, chop and place in the blender along with any other ingredients. The peel should only be removed from types of fruit that are inedible.

3. Now add some water and mix for about 15 seconds.

4. At the end add the rest of the water until the desired consistency is achieved and mix for another 5-10 seconds.

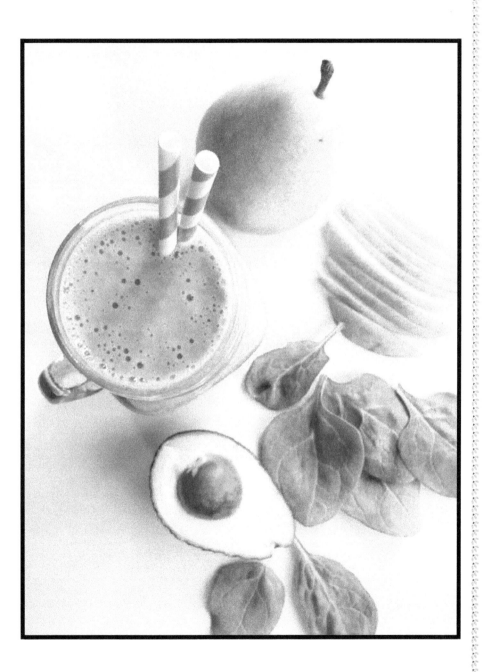

05_Spinach, Dandelion and Strawberries

Prep time: 5 minutes
Servings: 1-2

INGREDIENTS:

- **2** HANDFULS OF BABY SPINACH
- **1** SMALL HANDFUL OF DANDELIONS
- **150** G STRAWBERRIES
- **1** SMALL HANDFUL OF NETTLE
- SOME HONEY
- **150** ML OF WATER

DIRECTIONS:

1. Wash the vegetables, chop them roughly and put them in the blender first.

2. Then wash the fruit, remove the pits, chop and place in the blender along with any other ingredients. The peel should only be removed from types of fruit that are inedible.

3. Now add some water and mix for about 15 seconds.

4. At the end add the rest of the water until the desired consistency is achieved and mix for another 5-10 seconds.

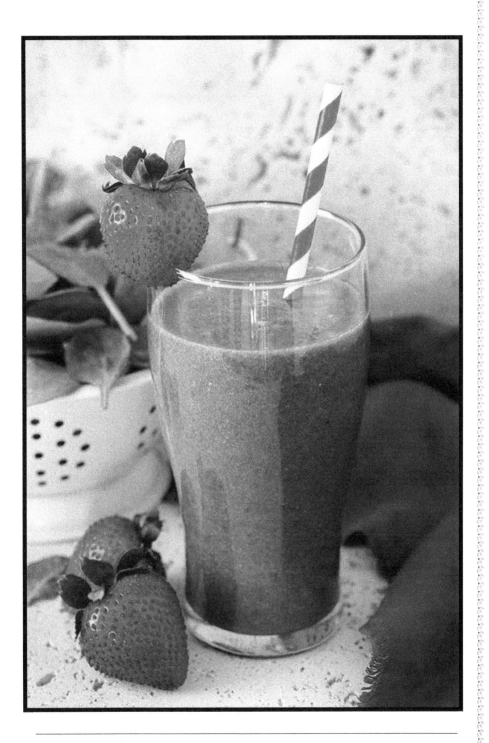

06_Spinach and Banana with Pineapple and Apple

Prep time: 5 minutes
Servings: 1-2

INGREDIENTS:

- **150** G SPINACH
- **1** MEDIUM-SIZED BANANA
- **100** G PINEAPPLE
- **1** SMALL APPLE

- **100-150** ML OF WATER

DIRECTIONS:

1. Wash the vegetables, chop them roughly and put them in the blender first.

2. Then wash the fruit, remove the pits, chop and place in the blender along with any other ingredients. The peel should only be removed from types of fruit that are inedible.

3. Now add some water and mix for about 15 seconds.

4. At the end add the rest of the water until the desired consistency is achieved and mix for another 5-10 seconds.

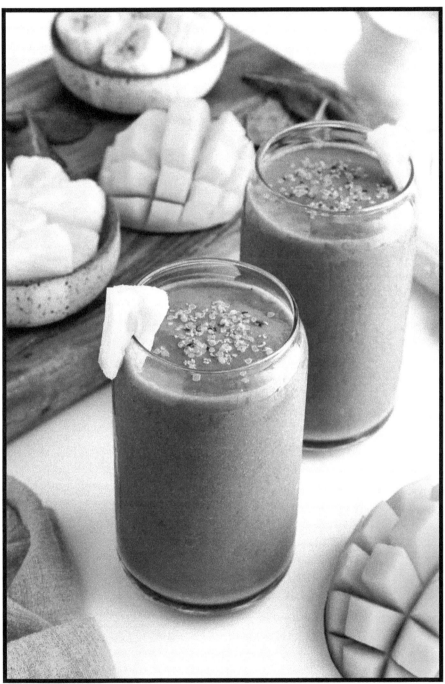

07_Spinach and Carrot with Blueberry, Pear and Banana

Prep time: 5 minutes
Servings: 1-2

INGREDIENTS:

- **150** G SPINACH
- **1** MEDIUM CARROT
- **50** G BLUEBERRIES
- **1** LARGE PEAR
- **1** SMALL BANANA
- **4-5** ICE CUBES
- JUICE OF **2** ORANGES
- **100-150** ML OF WATER

DIRECTIONS:

1. Wash the vegetables, chop them roughly and put them in the blender first.

2. Then wash the fruit, remove the pits, chop and place in the blender along with any other ingredients. The peel should only be removed from types of fruit that are inedible.

3. Now add the water and mix for about 15 seconds. Serve and enjoy.

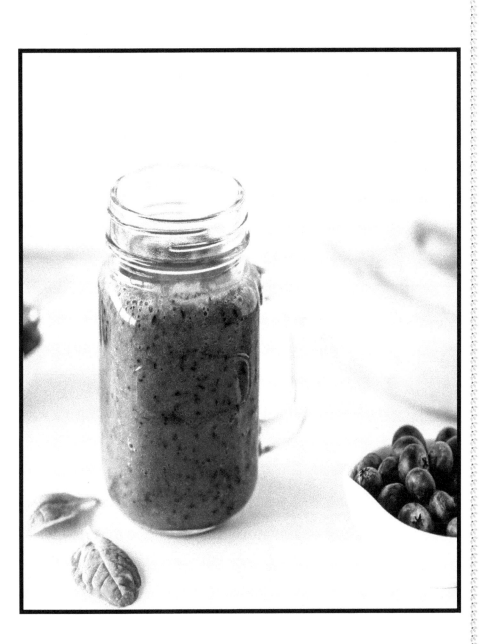

08_Spinach and Papaya with Pear

Prep time: 5 minutes
Servings: 1-2

INGREDIENTS:

- **2** HANDFULS OF SPINACH
- **200** G PAPAYA
- **1** LARGE PEAR
- **2** TBSP GOJI BERRIES (DRIED OR FRESH)
- **10** MINT LEAVES
- **250-300** ML WATER

DIRECTIONS:

1. Wash the vegetables, chop them roughly and put them in the blender first.

2. Then wash the fruit, remove the pits, chop and place in the blender along with any other ingredients. The peel should only be removed from types of fruit that are inedible.

3. Now add some water and mix for about 15 seconds.

4. At the end add the rest of the water until the desired consistency is achieved and mix for another 5-10 seconds.

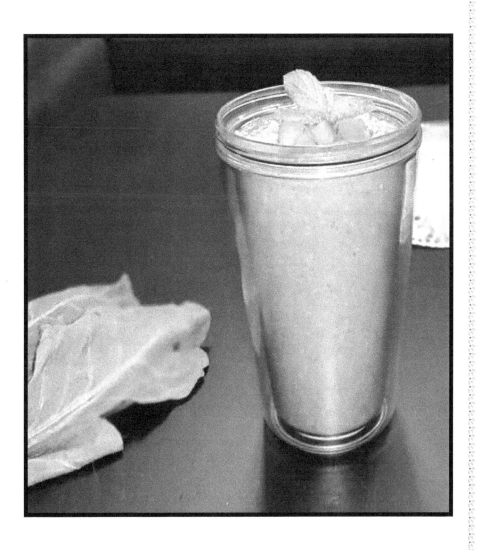

09_Spinach, Carrot, Celery and Blueberries

Prep time: 5 minutes
Servings: 1-2

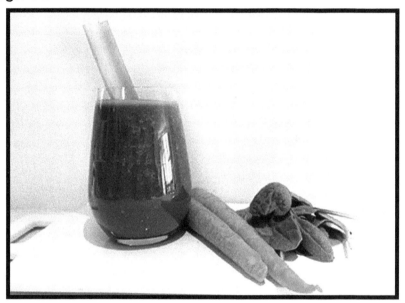

INGREDIENTS:

- **150** G SPINACH
- **1** SMALL CARROT
- **1** STICK OF CELERY
- **50** G BLUEBERRIES
- **1/2** MANGO
- **1** SMALL ORANGE
- **1** TBSP HONEY
- **200-250** ML OF WATER

DIRECTIONS AS A PREVIOUS RECIPE

10_Spinach and Cucumber with Pear and Avocado

Prep time: 5 minutes
Servings: 1-2

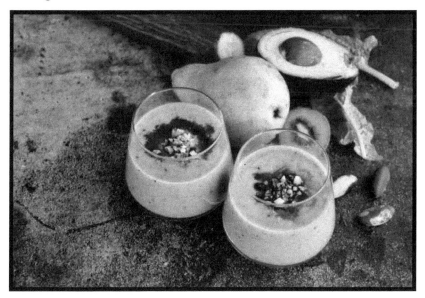

INGREDIENTS:

- 1 SMALL CUCUMBER
- 50 G SPINACH
- 1 MEDIUM PEAR
- 1/2 AVOCADO
- 2-3 MINT LEAVES
- 150-200 ML OF WATER

DIRECTIONS AS A NEXT RECIPE

11_Spinach, Pineapple and Avocado

Prep time: 5 minutes
Servings: 1-2

INGREDIENTS:

- **150** G. SPINACH
- **100** G. PINEAPPLE
- **1/4** AVOCADO
- JUICE OF **1** ORANGE

- **100-150** ML. WATER

DIRECTIONS:

1. Wash the vegetables, chop them roughly and put them in the blender first.

2. Then wash the fruit, remove the pits, chop and place in the blender along with any other ingredients. The peel should only be removed from types of fruit that are inedible.

3. Now add some water and mix for about 15 seconds.

4. At the end add the rest of the water until the desired consistency is achieved and mix for another 5-10 seconds.

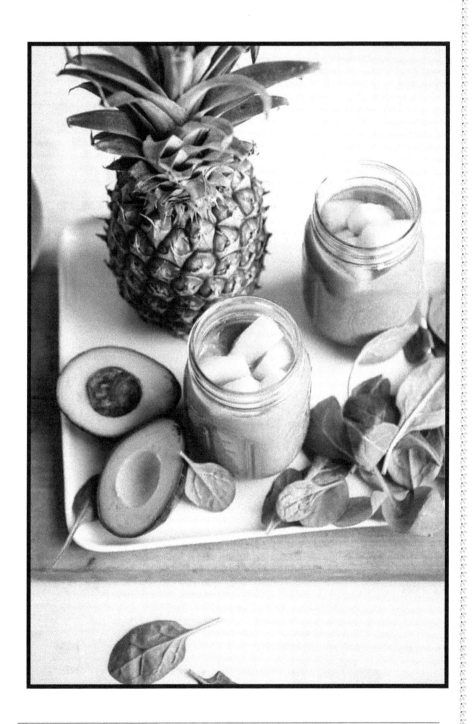

12_Lamb's Lettuce with Pear and Apple

Prep time: 5 minutes
Servings: 1-2

INGREDIENTS:

- **200** G LAMB'S LETTUCE
- **1** MEDIUM PEAR
- **1** MEDIUM APPLE
- **200-250** ML OF WATER

DIRECTIONS:

1. Wash the vegetables, chop them roughly and put them in the blender first.

2. Then wash the fruit, remove the pits, chop and place in the blender along with any other ingredients. The peel should only be removed from types of fruit that are inedible.

3. Now add some water and mix for about 15 seconds.

4. At the end add the rest of the water until the desired consistency is achieved and mix for another 5-10 seconds.

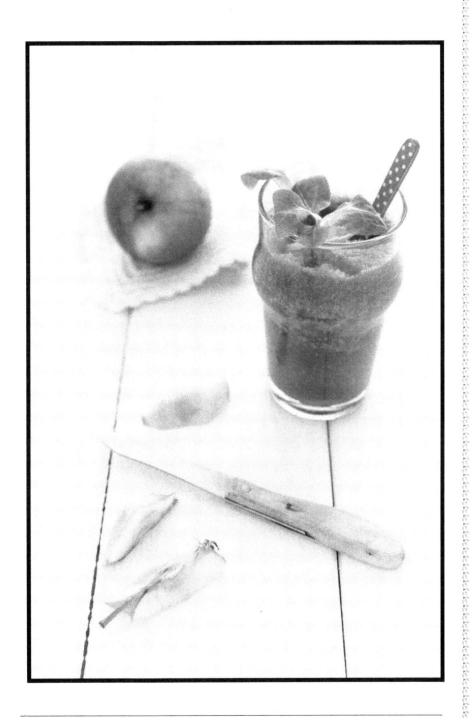

13_Corn Salad with Pineapple & Banana

Prep time: 5 minutes
Servings: 1-2

INGREDIENTS:

- **150** G LAMB'S LETTUCE
- **150** G PINEAPPLE
- **1** MEDIUM-SIZED BANANA
- **250-300** ML OF WATER

DIRECTIONS:

1. Wash the vegetables, chop them roughly and put them in the blender first.

2. Then wash the fruit, remove the pits, chop and place in the blender along with any other ingredients. The peel should only be removed from types of fruit that are inedible.

3. Now add some water and mix for about 15 seconds.

4. At the end add the rest of the water until the desired consistency is achieved and mix for another 5-10 seconds.

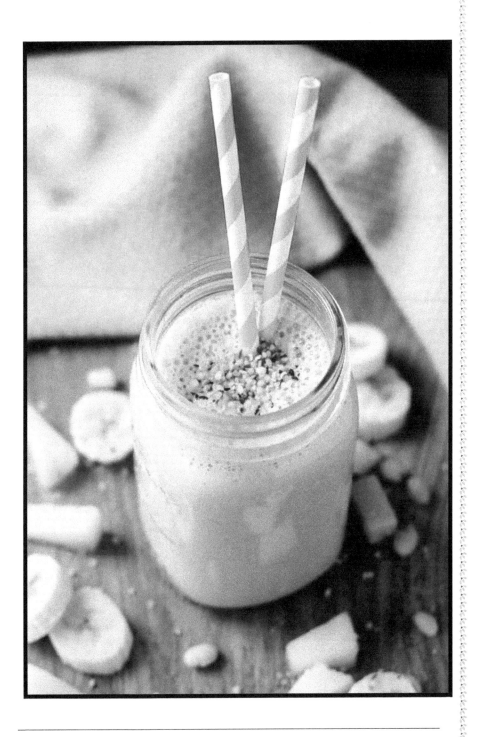

14_Lamb's Lettuce with Orange and Apple

Prep time: 5 minutes
Servings: 1-2

INGREDIENTS:

- **2** HANDFULS OF LAMB'S LETTUCE
- **1** ORANGE
- **1** APPLE
- **200-250** ML OF WATER

DIRECTIONS:

1. Wash the vegetables, chop them roughly and put them in the blender first.

2. Then wash the fruit, remove the pits, chop and place in the blender along with any other ingredients. The peel should only be removed from types of fruit that are inedible.

3. Now add some water and mix for about 15 seconds.

4. At the end add the rest of the water until the desired consistency is achieved and mix for another 5-10 seconds.

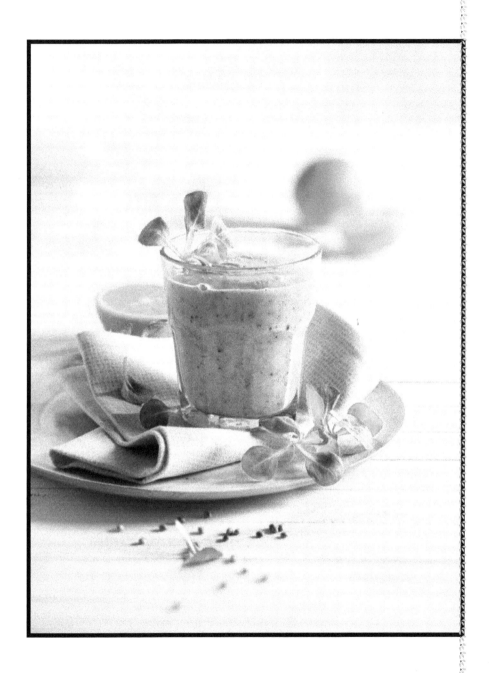

15_Lettuce with Apple and Banana

Prep time: 5 minutes
Servings: 1-2

INGREDIENTS:

- **200** G OF LETTUCE
- **1** LARGE APPLE
- **1** MEDIUM-SIZED BANANA
- **250-300** ML OF WATER

DIRECTIONS:

1. Wash the vegetables, chop them roughly and put them in the blender first.

2. Then wash the fruit, remove the pits, chop and place in the blender along with any other ingredients. The peel should only be removed from types of fruit that are inedible.

3. Now add some water and mix for about 15 seconds.

4. At the end add the rest of the water until the desired consistency is achieved and mix for another 5-10 seconds.

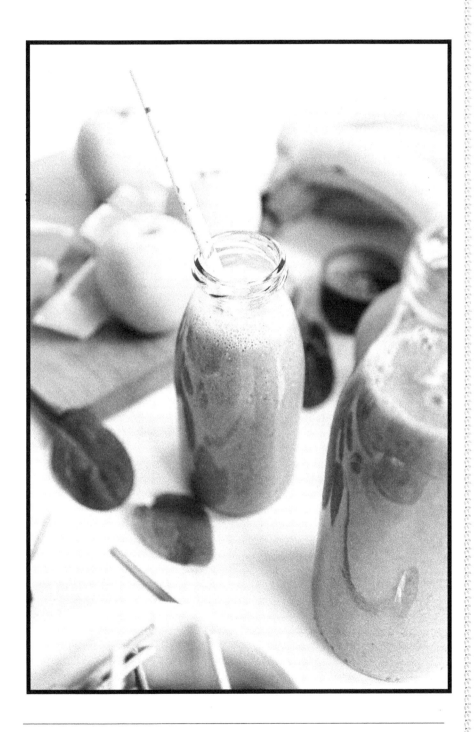

16_Kale with Orange and Apple

Prep time: 5 minutes
Servings: 1-2

INGREDIENTS:

- **150** G KALE
- JUICE OF **1** ORANGE
- **2** MEDIUM-SIZED APPLES
- JUICE OF **1** LEMON
- **100-150** ML OF WATER

DIRECTIONS:

1. Wash the vegetables, chop them roughly and put them in the blender first.

2. Then wash the fruit, remove the pits, chop and place in the blender along with any other ingredients. The peel should only be removed from types of fruit that are inedible.

3. Now add some water and mix for about 15 seconds.

4. At the end add the rest of the water until the desired consistency is achieved and mix for another 5-10 seconds.

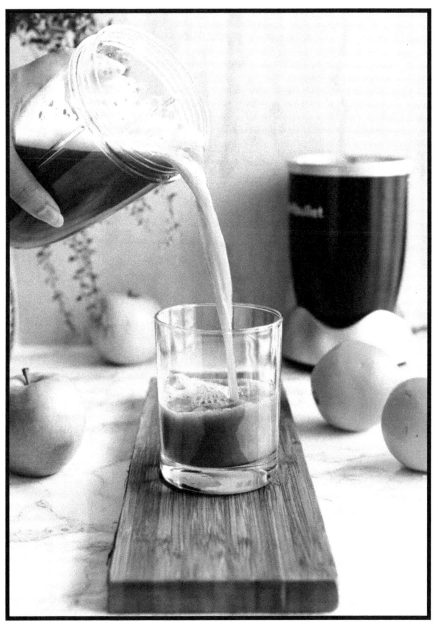

17_ Kale and Blackberry with Pineapple

Prep time: 5 minutes
Servings: 1-2

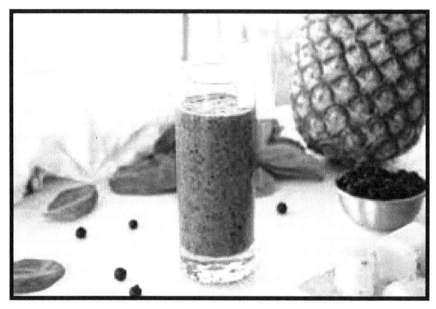

INGREDIENTS:

- 150 G KALE
- 50 G BLACKBERRIES
- 100 G PINEAPPLE
- 2 DRIED FIGS
- 1 TBSP VANILLA EXTRACT
- 200-250 ML OF WATER

DIRECTIONS AS NEXT PAGE

18_Kale, parsley, date and vanilla

Prep time: 5 minutes
Servings: 1-2

INGREDIENTS:

- **2** HANDFULS OF KALE
- **1** HANDFUL OF PARSLEY
- **2** DATES
- **1** APPLE
- **1** BANANA
- **1** PINCH OF CAYENNE PEPPER
- **1** PINCH OF VANILLA
- **300-350** ML OF WATER

DIRECTIONS:

1. Wash the vegetables, chop them roughly and put them in the blender first.

2. Then wash the fruit, remove the pits, chop and place in the blender along with any other ingredients. The peel should only be removed from types of fruit that are inedible.

3. Now add some water and mix for about 15 seconds.

4. At the end add the rest of the water until the desired consistency is achieved and mix for another 5-10 seconds.

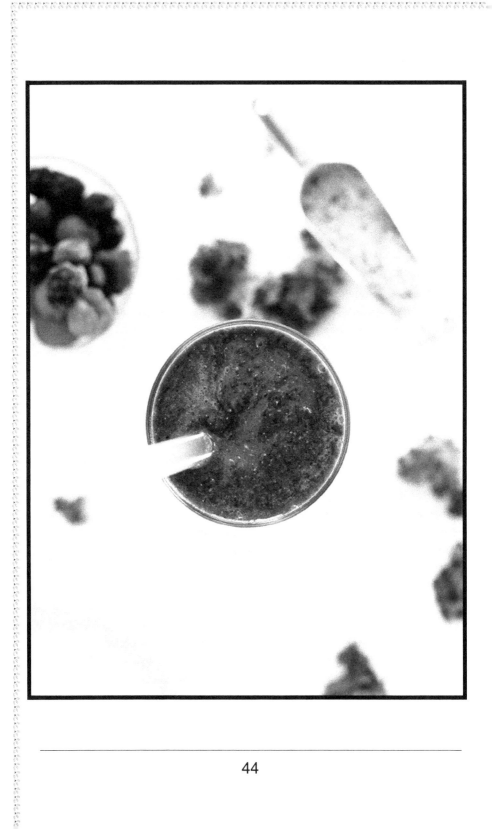

19_Kale, Orange with Raspberry and Banana

Prep time: 5 minutes
Servings: 1-2

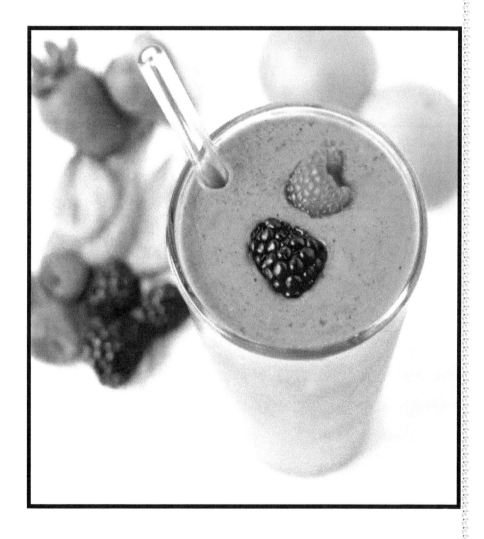

INGREDIENTS:

- **150** G KALE
- **1** ORANGE
- **100** G RASPBERRIES
- **1** SMALL BANANA
- **1** TEASPOON FLAXSEED
- **150-200** ML OF WATER

DIRECTIONS:

1. Wash the vegetables, chop them roughly and put them in the blender first.

2. Then wash the fruit remove the pits, chop and place in the blender along with any other ingredients. The peel should only be removed from types of fruit that are inedible.

3. Now add some water and mix for about 15 seconds.

4. At the end add the rest of the water until the desired consistency is achieved and mix for another 5-10 seconds.

20_Swiss chard-orange-carrot

Prep time: 5 minutes
Servings: 1-2

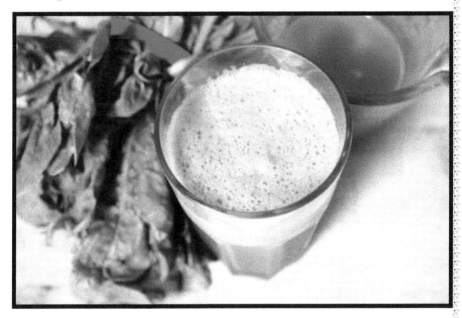

INGREDIENTS:

- 150 G SWISS CHARD
- 1 ORANGE
- 1 SMALL CARROT
- 2000-250 ML OF WATER

DIRECTIONS AS SIDE PAGE

21_Cucumber, Watermelon and Plum

Prep time: 5 minutes
Servings: 1-2

INGREDIENTS:

- **1** MEDIUM-SIZED CUCUMBER
- **100** G WATERMELON
- **2** PLUMS
- **100-150** ML OF WATER

DIRECTIONS:

1. Wash the vegetables, chop them roughly and put them in the blender first.

2. Then wash the fruit, remove the pits, chop and place in the blender along with any other ingredients. The peel should only be removed from types of fruit that are inedible.

3. Now add some water and mix for about 15 seconds.

4. At the end add the rest of the water until the desired consistency is achieved and mix for another 5-10 seconds.

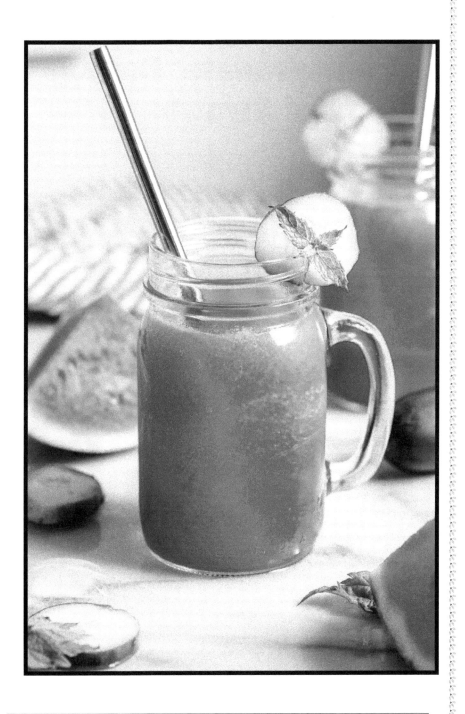

22_Cucumber, Pomegranate, Banana and Strawberry

Prep time: 5 minutes
Servings: 1-2

INGREDIENTS:

- **1** MEDIUM-SIZED CUCUMBER
- **1** POMEGRANATE
- **1** SMALL BANANA
- **5-6** STRAWBERRIES
- **1/8** TEASPOON OF GRATED NUTMEG
- **1/4** TEASPOON GROUND CLOVES
- **200-250** ML OF WATER

DIRECTIONS:

1. Wash the vegetables, chop them roughly and put them in the blender first.

2. Then wash the fruit, remove the pits, chop and place in the blender along with any other ingredients. The peel should only be removed from types of fruit that are inedible.

3. Now add some water and mix for about 15 seconds.

4. At the end add the rest of the water until the desired consistency is achieved and mix for another 5-10 seconds.

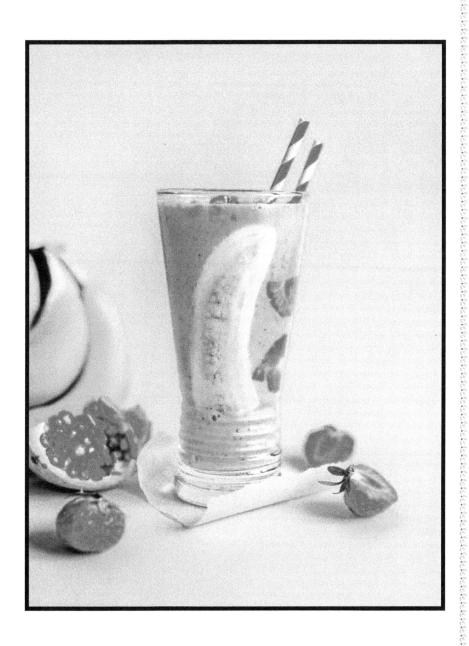

23_Cucumber, Parsley, Banana and Apple

Prep time: 5 minutes
Servings: 1-2

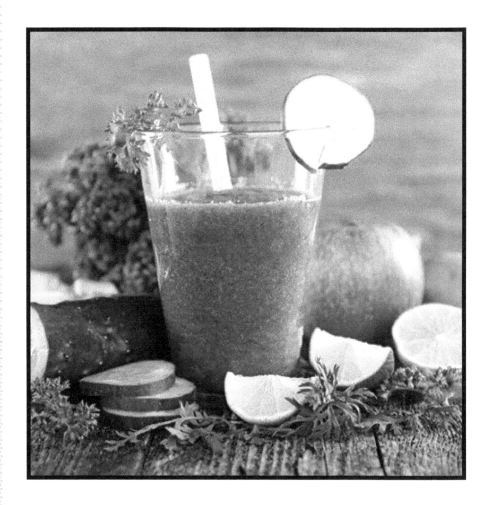

Ingredients:

- 1/2 CUCUMBER
- 1 BUNCH OF PARSLEY
- 1 BANANA
- 1 APPLE
- 200-250 ML OF WATER

Directions:

1. Wash the vegetables, chop them roughly and put them in the blender first.

2. Then wash the fruit, remove the pits, chop and place in the blender along with any other ingredients. The peel should only be removed from types of fruit that are inedible.

3. Now add some water and mix for about 15 seconds.

4. At the end add the rest of the water until the desired consistency is achieved and mix for another 5-10 seconds.

24_Cucumber with Coriander and Banana

Prep time: 5 minutes
Servings: 1-2

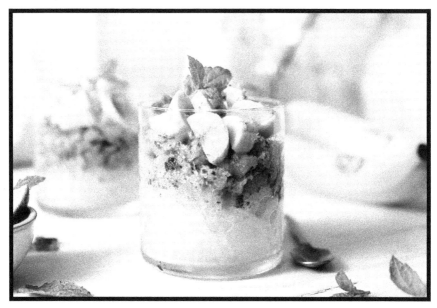

INGREDIENTS:

- **1** LARGE CUCUMBER
- **1** HANDFUL OF CORIANDER
- **1** MEDIUM-SIZED BANANA
- **1** BUNCH OF PARSLEY
- **200-250** ML OF WATER

DIRECTIONS AS PREVIOUS RECIPE

25_Cucumber, Lime and Tomato

Prep time: 5 minutes
Servings: 1-2

INGREDIENTS:

- **1** SMALL CUCUMBER
- **1** LIME
- **1** SMALL TOMATO
- **1/2** GREEN PEPPER
- **2** SPRIGS OF CORIANDER
- **150-200** ML OF WATER

DIRECTIONS:

1. Wash the vegetables, chop them roughly and put them in the blender first.

2. Then wash the fruit, remove the pits, chop and place in the blender along with any other ingredients. The peel should only be removed from types of fruit that are inedible.

3. Now add some water and mix for about 15 seconds.

4. At the end add the rest of the water until the desired consistency is achieved and mix for another 5-10 seconds.

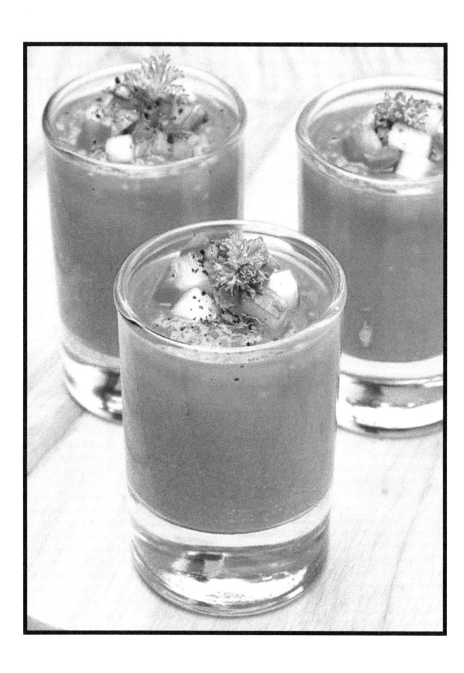

26_Celery, Lime and Orange

Prep time: 5 minutes
Servings: 1-2

INGREDIENTS:

- **2** STALKS OF CELERY
- **1/2** LIME
- **1** ORANGE
- **1** TEASPOON HORSERADISH
- **150-200** ML OF WATER

DIRECTIONS:

1. Wash the vegetables, chop them roughly and put them in the blender first.

2. Then wash the fruit, remove the pits, chop and place in the blender along with any other ingredients. The peel should only be removed from types of fruit that are inedible.

3. Now add some water and mix for about 15 seconds.

4. At the end add the rest of the water until the desired consistency is achieved and mix for another 5-10 seconds.

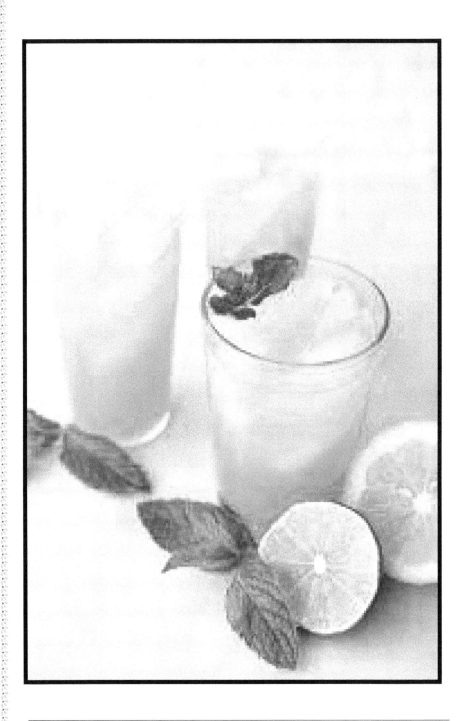

27_Celery, Papaya and Chard

Prep time: 5 minutes
Servings: 1-2

INGREDIENTS:

- **2** STALKS OF CELERY
- **1/2** PAPAYA
- **100** G SWISS CHARD
- **200-250** ML OF WATER

DIRECTIONS:

1. Wash the vegetables, chop them roughly and put them in the blender first.

2. Then wash the fruit, remove the pits, chop and place in the blender along with any other ingredients. The peel should only be removed from types of fruit that are inedible.

3. Now add some water and mix for about 15 seconds.

4. At the end add the rest of the water until the desired consistency is achieved and mix for another 5-10 seconds.

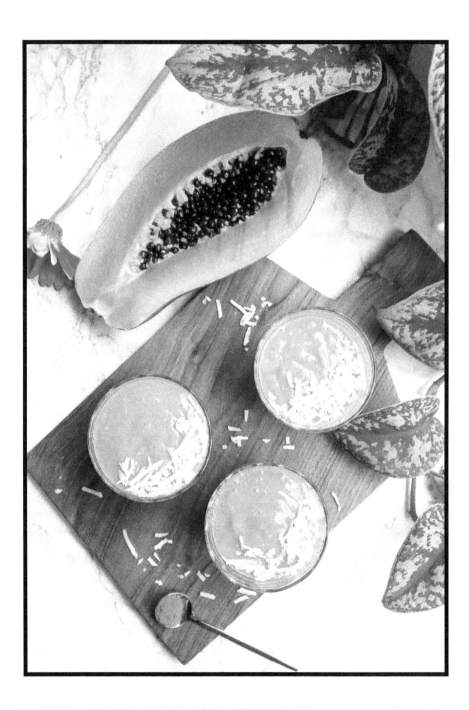

Chapter 3

FRUIT & VEGETABLE SMOOTHIES WITH MILK AND JUICES

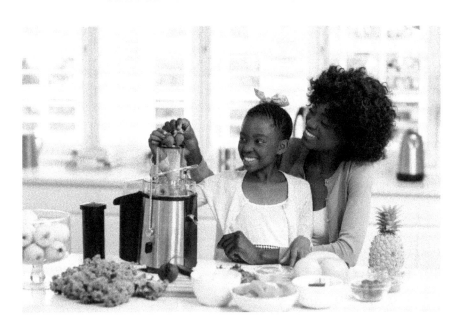

28_Spinach, Apple and Cucumber

Prep time: 5 minutes
Servings: 1-2

INGREDIENTS:

- **2** HANDFULS OF SPINACH
- **2** MEDIUM-SIZED APPLES
- **100** G CUCUMBER
- **4-5** ICE CUBES
- **1** TEASPOON HONEY
- **200-250** ML COCONUT MILK

DIRECTIONS:

1. Wash the vegetables, chop them roughly and put them in the blender first.

2. Then wash the fruit, remove the pits, chop and place in the blender along with any other ingredients. The peel should only be removed from types of fruit that are inedible.

3. Now add some coconut milk and mix for about 15 seconds.

4. At the end add the rest of the coconut milk until the desired consistency is achieved and mix for another 5-10 seconds.

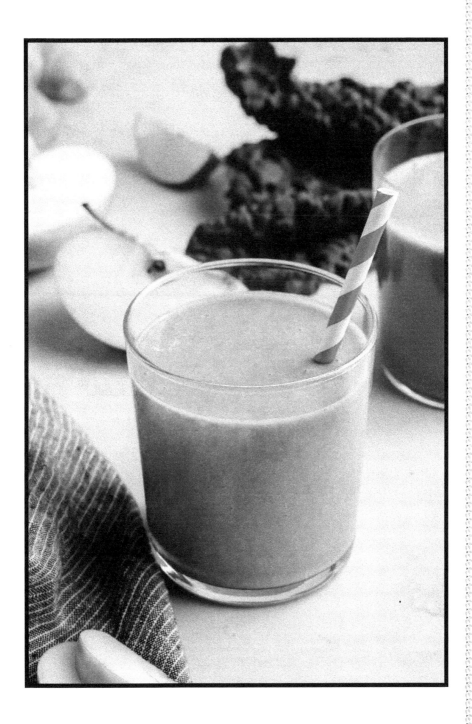

29_Spinach and Strawberry

Prep time: 5 minutes
Servings: 1-2

INGREDIENTS:

- **100** G SPINACH
- **3-4** LARGE STRAWBERRIES
- **3-4** ICE CUBES
- **150-200** ML COCONUT WATER

DIRECTIONS:

1. Wash the vegetables, chop them roughly and put them in the blender first.

2. Then wash the fruit, remove the pits, chop and place in the blender along with any other ingredients. The peel should only be removed from types of fruit that are inedible.

3. Now add some coconut water and mix for about 15 seconds.

4. At the end add the rest of the coconut water until the desired consistency is achieved and mix for another 5-10 seconds.

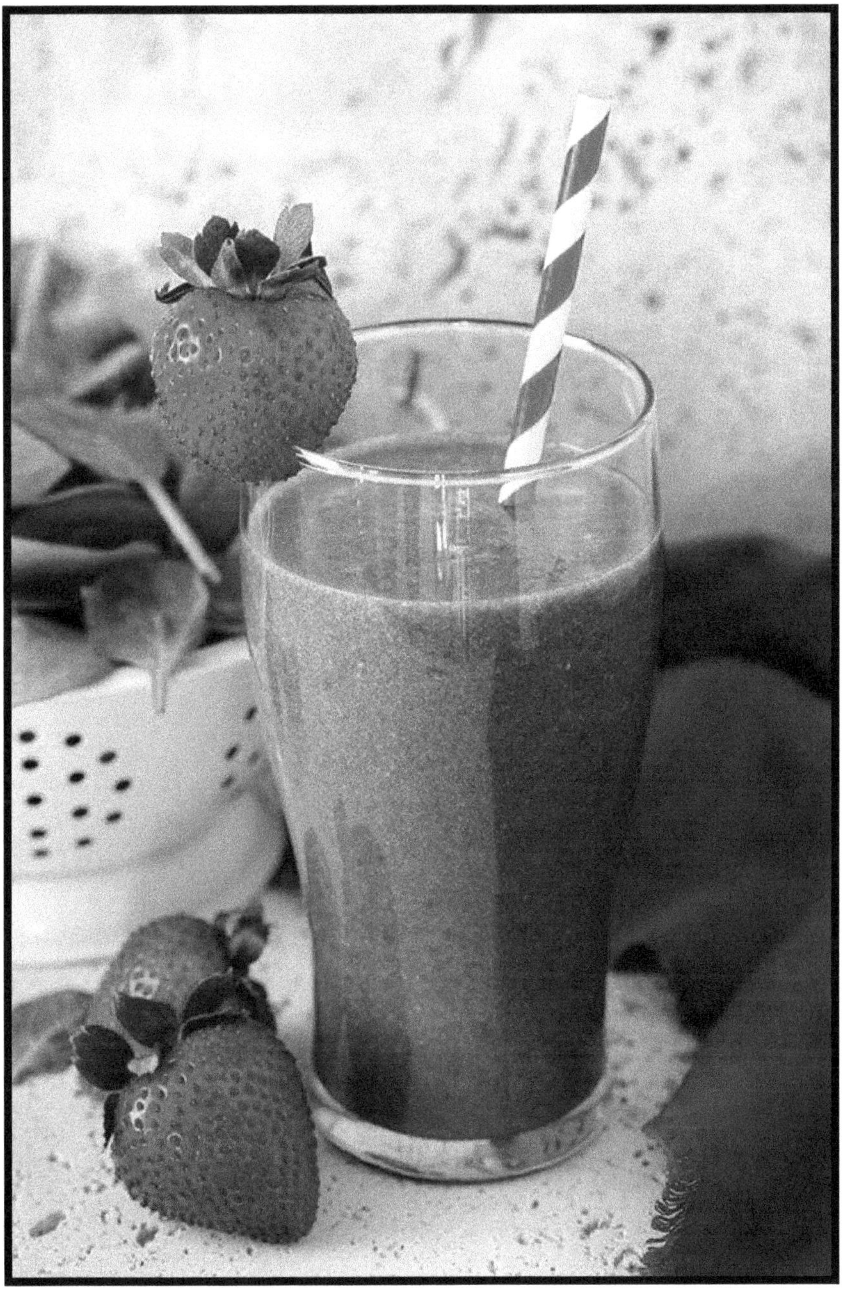

30_Spinach and Honeywith Avocado and Strawberries

Prep time: 5 minutes
Servings: 1-2

INGREDIENTS:

- **1** HANDFUL OF SPINACH
- **1/4** AVOCADO
- **1** TEASPOON HONEY
-
- **5-6** STRAWBERRIES
- **1** TEASPOON COCONUT OIL
- **1/4** TEASPOON CHILI POWDER
- **4-5** ICE CUBES
- **200** ML COCONUT MILK

DIRECTIONS AS RECIPE NR 33

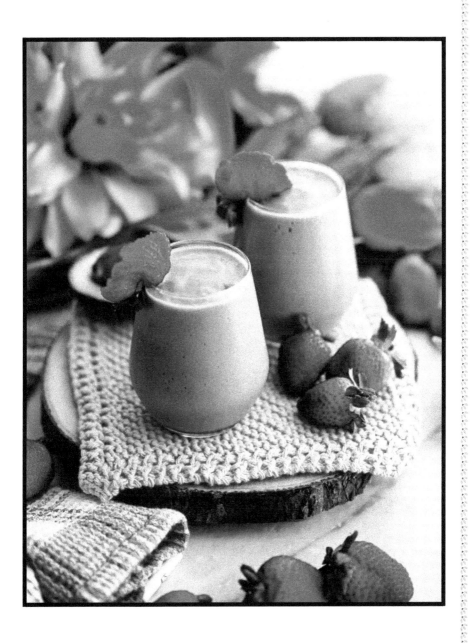

31_Spinach, Peppermint and Banana

Prep time: 5 minutes
Servings: 1-2

INGREDIENTS:

- **150** G SPINACH
- **1** TBSP PEPPERMINT EXTRACT
- **1** SMALL BANANA
- **2** TBSP COCOA POWDER WITHOUT SUGAR
- **1** TBSP CHIA SEEDS
- **4-5** ICE CUBES
- **250-300** ML ALMOND MILK

DIRECTIONS:

1. Wash the vegetables, chop them roughly and put them in the blender first.

2. Then wash the fruit, remove the pits, chop and place in the blender along with any other ingredients. The peel should only be removed from types of fruit that are inedible.

3. Now add some almond milk and mix for about 15 seconds.

4. At the end add the rest of the almond milk until the desired consistency is achieved and mix for another 5-10 seconds.

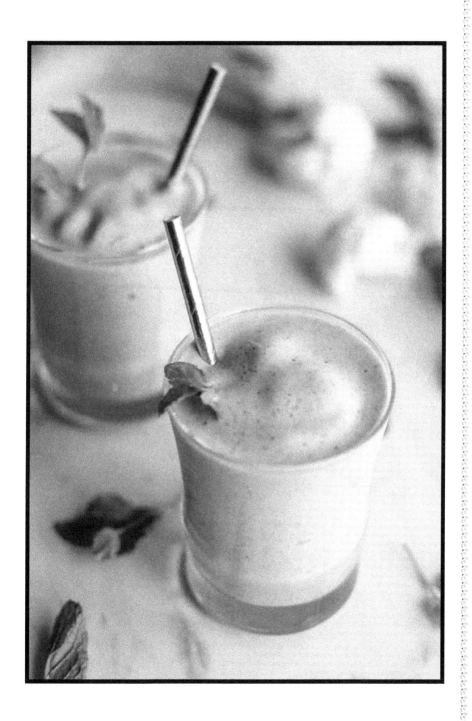

32_Spinach and Apricot with Avocado and Yogurt

Prep time: 5 minutes
Servings: 1-2

INGREDIENTS:

- **100** G SPINACH
- **1** APRICOT
- **1/2** AVOCADO
- **150** G GREEK YOGURT
- **1** TEASPOON HONEY
- **4-5** ICE CUBES
- **200-250** ML MILK (OR SOY MILK)

DIRECTIONS:

1. Wash the vegetables, chop them roughly and put them in the blender first.

2. Then wash the fruit, remove the pits, chop and place in the blender along with any other ingredients. The peel should only be removed from types of fruit that are inedible.

3. Now add some soy milk and mix for about 15 seconds.

4. At the end add the rest of the soy milk until the desired consistency is achieved and mix for another 5-10 seconds.

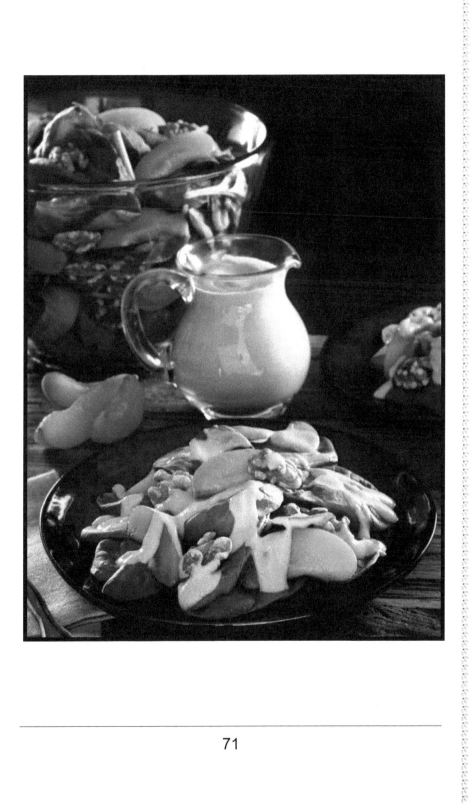

33_Spinach with Kale and Banana

Prep time: 5 minutes
Servings: 1-2

NGREDIENTS:

- **1** HANDFUL OF SPINACH
- **1** HANDFUL OF KALE
- **1** BANANA
- **1** TABLESPOON OF COCONUT OIL
- **50** ML ORANGE JUICE
- **100** ML ALMOND MILK

DIRECTIONS:

1. Wash the vegetables, chop them roughly and put them in the blender first.

2. Then wash the fruit, remove the pits, chop and place in the blender along with any other ingredients. The peel should only be removed from types of fruit that are inedible.

3. Now add some almond milk and mix for about 15 seconds.

4. At the end add the rest of the almond milk until the desired consistency is achieved and mix for another 5-10 seconds.

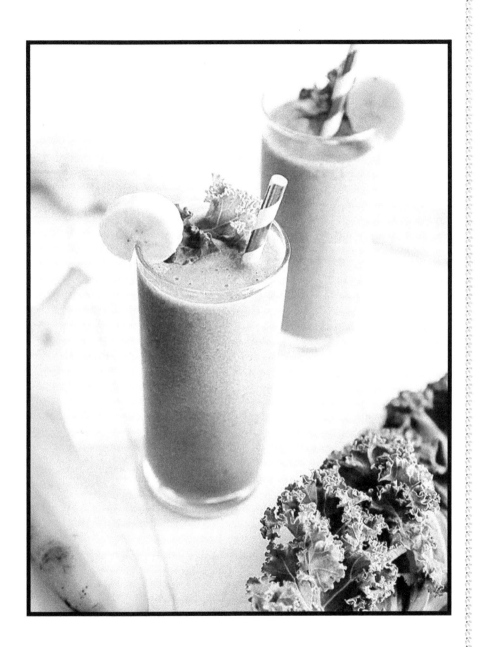

34_Lamb's Lettuce with Apricot and Peach

Prep time: 5 minutes

Servings: 1-2

INGREDIENTS:

- **150** G LAMB'S LETTUCE
- **1** APRICOT
- **1** PEACH
- **150-200** ML COCONUT MILK

DIRECTIONS:

1. Wash the vegetables, chop them roughly and put them in the blender first.

2. Then wash the fruit, remove the pits, chop and place in the blender along with any other ingredients. The peel should only be removed from types of fruit that are inedible.

3. Now add some coconut milk and mix for about 15 seconds.

4. At the end add the rest of the coconut milk until the desired consistency is achieved and mix for another 5-10 seconds.

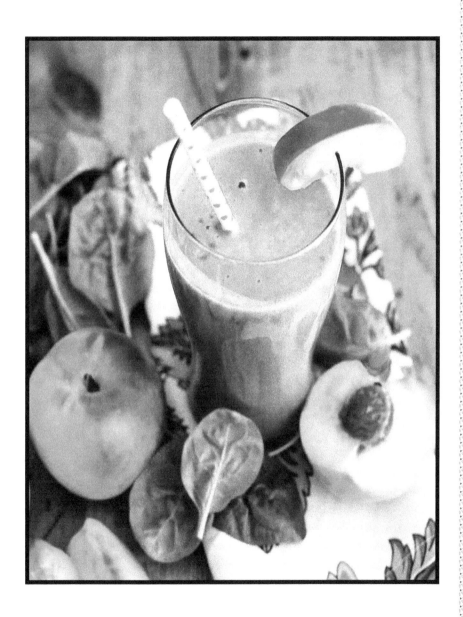

35_Lettuce, Banana, Yogurt and Cinnamon

Prep time: 5 minutes
Servings: 1-2

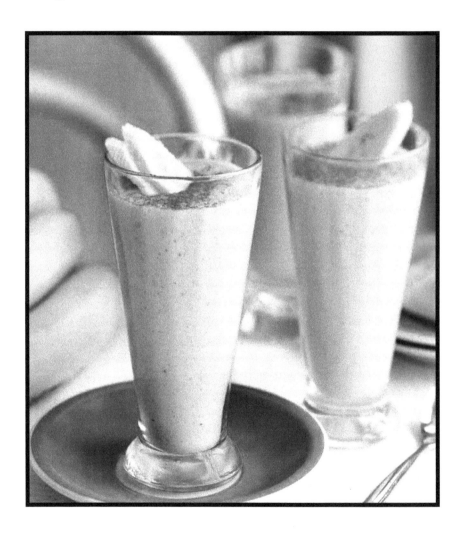

INGREDIENTS:

- **2** HANDFULS OF LETTUCE
- **1** BANANA
- **150** G LOW-FAT YOGURT
- **1** PINCH OF CINNAMON
- **3-4** ICE CUBES
- **200** ML ALMOND MILK

DIRECTIONS:

1. Wash the vegetables, chop them roughly and put them in the blender first.

2. Then wash the fruit, remove the pits, chop and place in the blender along with any other ingredients. The peel should only be removed from types of fruit that are inedible.

3. Now add some almond milk and mix for about 15 seconds.

4. At the end add the rest of the almond milk until the desired consistency is achieved and mix for another 5-10 seconds.

36_Kale and Almond butter with Banana

Prep time: 5 minutes
Servings: 1-2

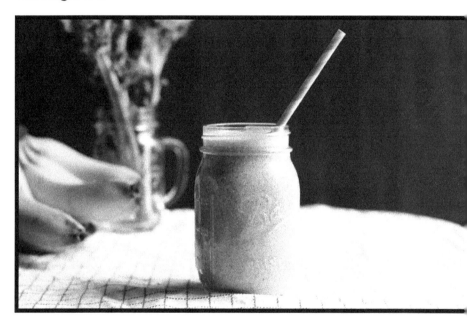

INGREDIENTS:

- 150 G. KALE
- 2 TEASPOONS OF ALMOND BUTTER
- 1 SMALL BANANA
- 1/8 TEASPOON CINNAMON
- 1/8 TEASPOON GROUND GINGER
- 200-250 ML ALMOND MILK

DIRECTIONS AS PREVIOUS RECIPE

37_Kale and Raspberry with Strawberry

Prep time: 5 minutes
Servings: 1-2

INGREDIENTS:

- **200** G KALE
- **100** G RASPBERRIES
- **100** G STRAWBERRIES
- **200-250** ML ALMOND MILK
-

DIRECTIONS:

1. Wash the vegetables, chop them roughly and put them in the blender first.

2. Then wash the fruit, remove the pits, chop and place in the blender along with any other ingredients. The peel should only be removed from types of fruit that are inedible.

3. Now add some almond milk and mix for about 15 seconds.

4. At the end add the rest of the almond milk until the desired consistency is achieved and mix for another 5-10 seconds.

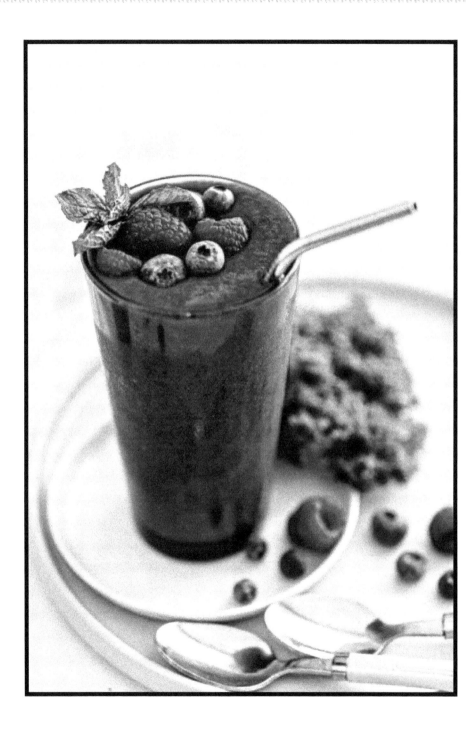

38_Swiss Chard and Blueberry with Raspberry

Prep time: 5 minutes
Servings: 1-2

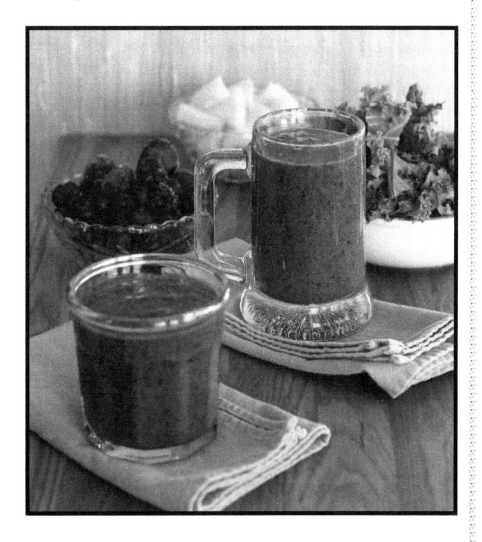

INGREDIENTS:

- 150 G SWISS CHARD
- 50 G BLUEBERRIES
- 50 G RASPBERRIES
- 150-200 ML COCONUT MILK

DIRECTIONS:

1. Wash the vegetables, chop them roughly and put them in the blender first.

2. Then wash the fruit, remove the pits, chop and place in the blender along with any other ingredients. The peel should only be removed from types of fruit that are inedible.

3. Now add some coconut milk and mix for about 15 seconds.

4. At the end add the rest of the coconut milk until the desired consistency is achieved and mix for another 5-10 seconds.

39_Cucumber, Orange and Fennel

Prep time: 5 minutes
Servings: 1-2

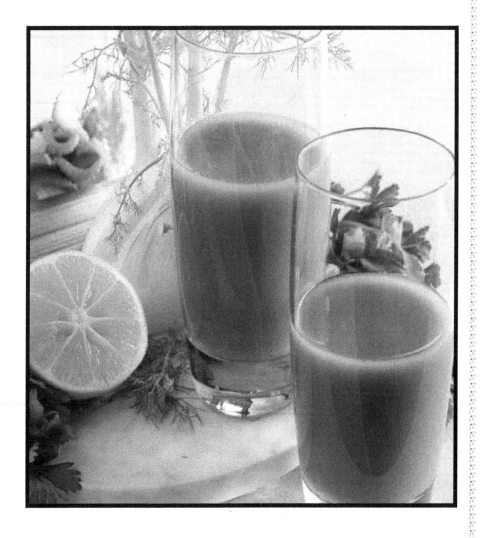

INGREDIENTS:

- **1** SMALL CUCUMBER
- **2** ORANGES
- **100** G FENNEL
- **2** TBSP LIME JUICE
- **150-200** ML COCONUT WATER

DIRECTIONS:

1. Wash the vegetables, chop them roughly and put them in the blender first.

2. Then wash the fruit, remove the pits, chop and place in the blender along with any other ingredients. The peel should only be removed from types of fruit that are inedible.

3. Now add some coconut water and mix for about 15 seconds.

4. At the end add the rest of the coconut water until the desired consistency is achieved and mix for another 5-10 seconds.

40_Cucumber with Yogurt and Kiwi

Prep time: 5 minutes
Servings: 1-2

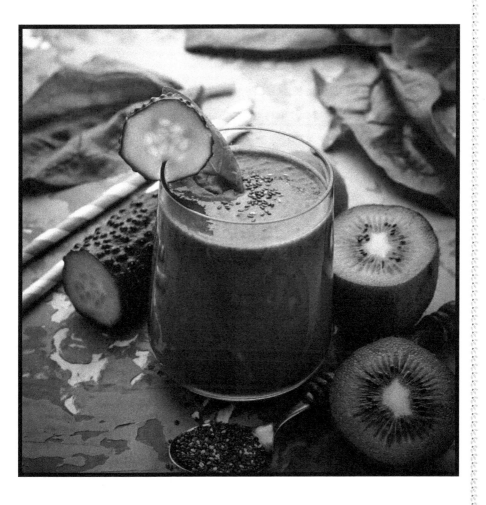

Ingredients:

- **1** MEDIUM-SIZED CUCUMBER
- **125-150** G YOGURT
- **2** KIWIS
- JUICE OF **1** LEMON
- **1** TBSP HONEY
- **1** TBSP CHIA SEEDS
- **2-3** ICE CUBES
- **200-250** ML ALMOND MILK

Directions:

1. Wash the vegetables, chop them roughly and put them in the blender first.

2. Then wash the fruit, remove the pits, chop and place in the blender along with any other ingredients. The peel should only be removed from types of fruit that are inedible.

3. Now add some almond milk and mix for about 15 seconds.

4. At the end add the rest of the almond milk until the desired consistency is achieved and mix for another 5-10 seconds.

41_Green Pepper with Celery and apple

Prep time: 5 minutes
Servings: 1-2

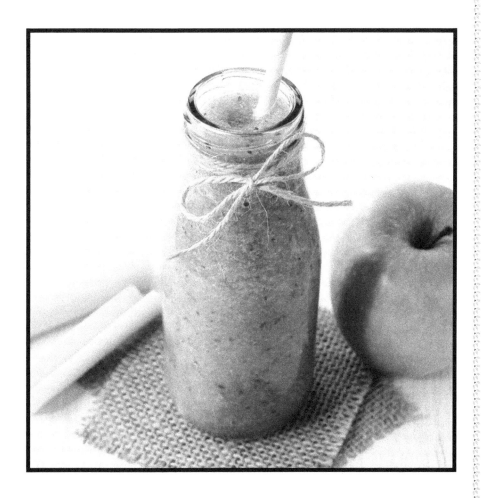

INGREDIENTS:

- **2** STALKS OF CELERY
- **2** MEDIUM-SIZED APPLES
- **1** GREEN PEPPER
- **250-300** ML APPLE JUICE

DIRECTIONS:

1. Wash the vegetables, chop them roughly and put them in the blender first.

2. Then wash the fruit, remove the pits, chop and place in the blender along with any other ingredients. The peel should only be removed from types of fruit that are inedible.

3. Now add some apple juice and mix for about 15 seconds.

4. At the end add the rest of the apple juice until the desired consistency is achieved and mix for another 5-10 seconds.

42_Avocado and Walnut, with Kale and Blueberry

Prep time: 5 minutes
Servings: 1-2

INGREDIENTS:

- 1/2 AVOCADO
- 5 WALNUTS
- 100 G KALE
- 50 G BLUEBERRIES
- 250-300 ML ALMOND MILK

DIRECTIONS:

1. Wash the vegetables, chop them roughly and put them in the blender first.

2. Then wash the fruit, remove the pits, chop and place in the blender along with any other ingredients. The peel should only be removed from types of fruit that are inedible.

3. Now add some almond milk and mix for about 15 seconds.

4. At the end add the rest of the almond milk until the desired consistency is achieved and mix for another 5-10 seconds.

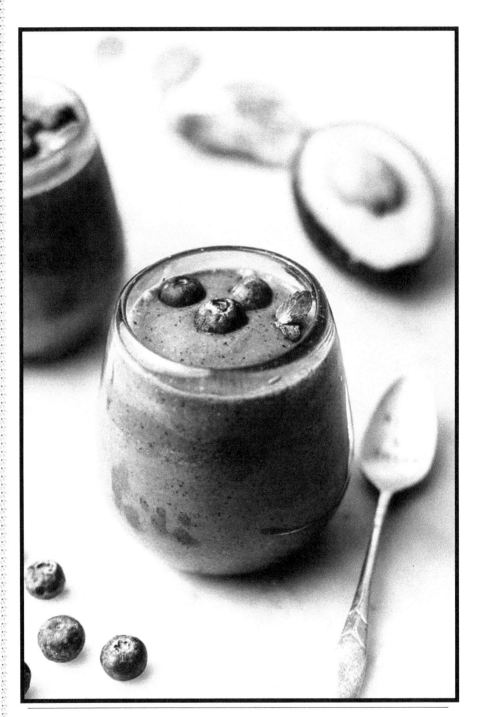

43_Avocado with Pumpkin Seed and Banana

Prep time: 5 minutes
Servings: 1-2

INGREDIENTS:

- 1/2 AVOCADO
- 1 TEASPOON. PUMPKIN SEEDS
- 1 SMALL BANANA
- 200-250 ML ALMOND MILK

DIRECTIONS:

1. Wash the vegetables, chop them roughly and put them in the blender first.

2. Then wash the fruit, remove the pits, chop and place in the blender along with any other ingredients. The peel should only be removed from types of fruit that are inedible.

3. Now add some almond milk and mix for about 15 seconds.

4. At the end add the rest of the almond milk until the desired consistency is achieved and mix for another 5-10 seconds.

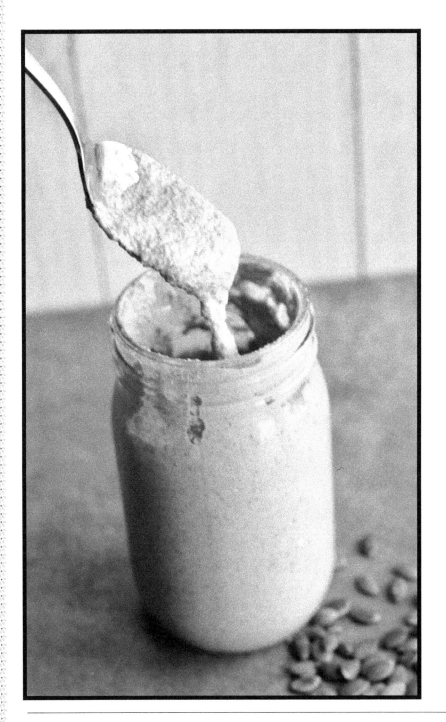

44_Avocado, Pineapple and Orange

Prep time: 5 minutes
Servings: 1-2

INGREDIENTS:

- **1** HALF AVOCADO
- **50** GRAMS OF PINEAPPLE
- **1** HANDFUL OF ENDIVE SALAD
- **1** HANDFUL OF WINTER PURSLANE
- **1** SMALL HANDFUL OF PARSLEY
- **1** TEASPOON HONEY
- JUICE OF ONE ORANGE
- **150** ML APPLE TEA

DIRECTIONS:

1. Wash the vegetables, chop them roughly and put them in the blender first.

2. Then wash the fruit, remove the pits, chop and place in the blender along with any other ingredients. The peel should only be removed from types of fruit that are inedible.

3. Now add the apple tea and mix for about 15 seconds. Serve and Enjoy

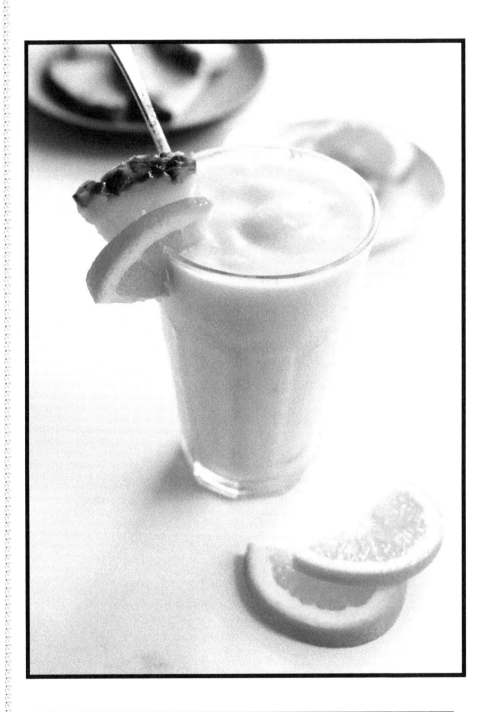

45_Avocado with Flax Seed and Blueberry

Prep time: 5 minutes
Servings: 1-2

INGREDIENTS:

- **1/2** AVOCADO
- **1** TBSP FLAXSEED
- **100** G BLUEBERRIES
- **1** TBSP COCOA POWDER
- **250-300** ML COCONUT WATER

DIRECTIONS:

1. Wash the vegetables, chop them roughly and put them in the blender first.

2. Then wash the fruit, remove the pits, chop and place in the blender along with any other ingredients. The peel should only be removed from types of fruit that are inedible.

3. Now add some coconut water and mix for about 15 seconds.

4. At the end add the rest of the coconut water until the desired consistency is achieved and mix for another 5-10 seconds.

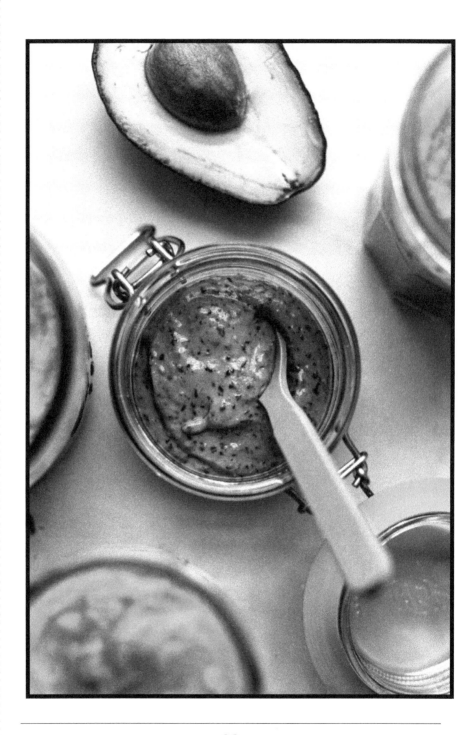

46_Avocado, Apricot and Peach

Prep time: 5 minutes
Servings: 1-2

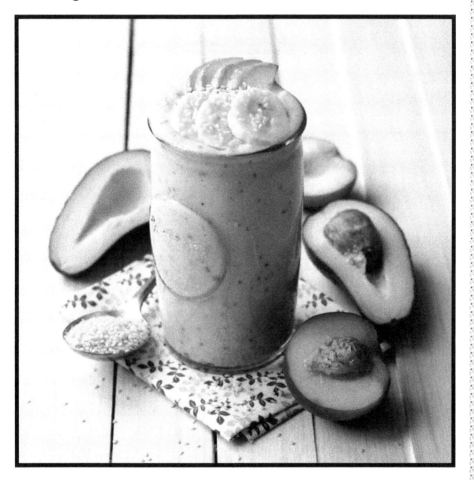

INGREDIENTS:

- **1** AVOCADO
- **2** APRICOTS
- **2** PEACHES
- **50** G ROSE HIPS
- **200-250** ML RICE MILK

DIRECTIONS:

1. Wash the vegetables, chop them roughly and put them in the blender first.

2. Then wash the fruit, remove the pits, chop and place in the blender along with any other ingredients. The peel should only be removed from types of fruit that are inedible.

3. Now add some lrice milk and mix for about 15 seconds.

4. At the end add the rest of the rice milk until the desired consistency is achieved and mix for another 5-10 seconds.

CONCLUSION

Nutritional values of ingredients

Aloe vera
Vitamins: A, B1, B2, B3, B6, B9, B12, C, E.
Minerals: calcium, iron, phosphorus, potassium, magnesium, sodium, copper and zinc.
Strengthens the immune system and aids digestion.

Pineapple
Vitamins: B3, B5, C, E.
Minerals: potassium, calcium, iron, magnesium, zinc.

Apple
Vitamins: A and C.
Minerals: potassium, iron, calcium. Magnesium.

Apricot
Vitamins: A, B1, B2, C.
Minerals: potassium, calcium, phosphorus.

Avocado
Vitamins: A, B, E
Minerals: calcium, potassium, magnesium.

Banana
Vitamins: B, C, E,
Minerals: sodium, calcium, potassium, magnesium, zinc, iron.

Pear
Vitamins: B and C.
Minerals: potassium, magnesium, calcium, phosphorus, zinc, copper.

Blueberry
Vitamins: B, C, E, carotenoids (provitamin A).
Minerals: iron, calcium, phosphorus, potassium, zinc,

manganese.

Blackberry

Vitamins : A, B3, B5, C, E, K.

Minerals : potassium, calcium, phosphorus, magnesium, iron, zinc.

Chia seeds

Above-average rich in antioxidants, proteins, fiber, vitamins (A, B1, B3, E) and minerals (calcium, iron, magnesium, potassium, boron, zinc).

They still have the highest omega-3 levels ever (over 18 grams per 100 grams - 10 times more than salmon). According to a study by the Nutritional Science Research Institute (Massachusetts, USA), chia seeds have a natural blood-thinning effect that significantly lowers the risk of a stroke or heart attack.

The study also came to the conclusion that chia seeds have a positive effect on blood sugar levels and can regulate them.

Clementine

Vitamins : A and C.

Minerals : potassium, sodium, calcium, magnesium, iron.

Date

Vitamin:B .

Minerals : iron, calcium, magnesium, phosphorus, potassium.

Strawberry

Vitamins : A and C.

Minerals : calcium, iron, zinc.

Coward

Vitamins : B1 and B2.

Minerals : calcium, potassium, iron, zinc.

Lamb's lettuce

Vitamins : A and C.
Minerals : calcium, phosphorus, sodium, iron, potassium.

Fennel
Vitamins : A and C.
Minerals : potassium, calcium, sulfur, phosphorus, magnesium, iron, zinc.
Has an expectorant effect, helps against coughs and runny nose.

Barley grass
Vitamins : B1 and C.
Minerals : calcium, iron, zinc. Lowers cholesterol levels.
Has a deacidifying effect, promotes digestion.

Goji berry
Vitamins : beta carotene (provitamin A), B1, B2, B3, C, E.
Minerals : sodium, magnesium, calcium, potassium and iron.
Strengthens the immune system, has a positive effect on the intestinal flora,
lowers the cholesterol level.

Pomegranate
Vitamins : A, B, C, E.
Minerals : calcium, potassium, magnesium, phosphorus, iron, copper, manganese.

Grapefruit
Vitamins : A, C, E.
Minerals : sodium, potassium, magnesium, calcium, iron, zinc

Kale
Vitamins : A, B6, C, K.
Minerals : calcium, magnesium, iron.

Cucumber
Vitamins : A, B1, C.
Minerals : calcium, zinc, iron, magnesium, potassium and

phosphorus.

Rose hip

Vitamins : A, B6, C.

Minerals : calcium, magnesium, iron.

Strengthens the immune system, lowers the cholesterol level, helps against colds.

Hemp seeds

Vitamins : A, B, C, D, E.

Minerals : calcium, potassium, magnesium, sulfur and iron.

Omega-3 and omega-6 fatty acids, gamma-linolenic acid and many antioxidants.

Strengthens the immune system, has anti-inflammatory effects, promotes metabolism.

Raspberry

Vitamins : B and C.

Minerals : potassium, calcium, magnesium, iron, manganese.

Honey

Has an anti-bacterial effect, helps with colds, coughs, sore throats and hoarseness.

Honeydew melon

Vitamins : B1, B2, B6, C, E.

Minerals : sodium, potassium, calcium, magnesium, iron, zinc.

Ginger

Vitamins : B6 and C.

Minerals : magnesium, calcium, iron.

Strengthens the immune system, protects the gastrointestinal function, promotes fat burning, anti-inflammatory, lowers blood pressure, stimulates digestion, helps against coughs.

Yogurt
Vitamins : A and B6.
Minerals : potassium, calcium, sodium, magnesium.

Currant
Vitamins : A, B2, B6, C, K.
Minerals : potassium, calcium, magnesium, iron.

Carrot
Vitamins : A, B, C, E.
Minerals : potassium, sodium, phosphorus, calcium, magnesium, zinc, iron.

Cherries
Vitamins : A, B1, B2, C, E.
Minerals : potassium, phosphorus, calcium, magnesium, sodium.

Kiwi
Vitamins : B, C, E.
Minerals : magnesium, phosphorus, potassium, calcium, iron.

Coconut milk
Vitamins : B1, B2, B3, B4, E, C.
Minerals : sodium, potassium, calcium, phosphorus, magnesium, iron, zinc, manganese and copper.

Coconut water
Vitamins : B1, B2, B3, B5, B6, B7, B9, C.
Minerals : calcium, potassium, magnesium, sodium, phosphorus, iron, copper, manganese and zinc.

Lettuce
Vitamins : A, B1, B2, C.
Minerals : sodium, magnesium, phosphorus, calcium, potassium, iron.

Linseed
High proportion of omega3 fatty acids.

Vitamins : B1, B6, E.
Minerals : copper, manganese, magnesium, phosphorus, selenium.
Strengthens the cardiovascular system, helps with high blood pressure, has anti-inflammatory effects, lowers cholesterol, promotes digestion, protects the liver, regulates blood sugar levels.

Lime
Vitamins : B1, B2, B6, C, E, beta-carotene (provitamin A).
Minerals : calcium, magnesium, iron, zinc.

Dandelion
Vitamins : beta-carotene (provitamin A), C, K.
Minerals : potassium, calcium, manganese, iron.
Strongly diuretic, has a dehydrating effect and lowers blood pressure.

Almond milk
Vitamins : B1, B3, B5, B6, B9, C, E, K.
Minerals : magnesium, calcium, iron, potassium,zinc,phosphorus.
Almond milk is lactose-free and therefore suitable for people with a lactose intolerance.

Mango
Vitamins : B1, B6, C, E.
Minerals : magnesium, potassium, calcium, manganese, zinc.

Swiss chard
Vitamins : A, B1, B2, C.
Minerals : potassium, calcium, magnesium, iron.

Matcha
Vitamins : A, B, E, C.
Minerals : potassium, calcium, iron.
Stimulates the metabolism, improves physical endurance, supports fat loss, promotes responsiveness and strengthens

the immune system and the defense cells.

Milk

Vitamins : A, B1, B2, B6, B12, D, E, K.

Minerals : calcium, iron, potassium, magnesium.

Mirabelle

Vitamins : A, B1, B2, B3, C.

Minerals : potassium, phosphorus, magnesium, calcium, iron, sodium.

Nectarine

Vitamins : B, C, E, beta-carotene (provitamin A).

Minerals : sodium, potassium, calcium, magnesium, iron, zinc.

Olive oil

Rich in monounsaturated fatty acids and polyphenols.Lowerscholesterol, strengthens the cardiovascular system and has an anti-aging effect.

Orange

Vitamins : C B.

Minerals : potassium, magnesium, calcium.

Papaya

Vitamins : A, C.

Minerals : magnesium, potassium, calcium, sodium.

Parsley

Vitamins : A, C, K, beta carotene (provitamin A).

Minerals : calcium, magnesium, phosphorus, iron, manganese, potassium.

Peach

Vitamins : A, B1, B2, C, E.

Minerals : potassium, calcium, phosphorus, magnesium.

Plum

Vitamins : B, C, E.

Minerals : iron, magnesium, potassium, copper, zinc.

Cranberry
Vitamins : beta carotene (provitamin A), B1, B2, B6, C, E.
Minerals : potassium, calcium, magnesium, phosphorus.

Rice milk
Lactose-free, therefore suitable for people with a lactose intolerance.
Can be used as a milk substitute in a vegan diet, but is very low in vitamins and minerals.

Beetroot
Vitamins : B1, B2, B6, C.
Minerals : potassium, calcium, iron, copper, magnesium, manganese, phosphorus, zinc.

Arugula
Vitamins : A, C.
Minerals : iron, calcium, potassium.

Sorrel
Vitamin:C .
Minerals : potassium, magnesium, iron.
Strengthens the immune system, lowers blood pressure and stimulates digestion. People with kidney disease, arthritis, gout or rheumatism should refrain from consuming it.

Celery
Vitamins : B1, B2, B12, C, E.
Minerals : calcium, iron, potassium.

Soy milk
Serves as a milk substitute in a vegan diet. Soy milk is definitely healthier than cow's milk for people with a very high blood fat level or who are lactose intolerant because it contains neither cholesterol nor lactose.
Contains less vitamin B2 and calcium than cow's milk.
Vitamin B12 is completely absent.

Spinach
Vitamins : C, beta carotene (provitamin A).
Minerals : iron, magnesium, potassium.

Ribwort plantain
Vitamin C .
Minerals : potassium, zinc.
Has anti-inflammatory, antibacterial, diuretic effects.
Helps with inflammation in the mouth and throat. Particularly suitable
against coughing.

Stevia
Contains neither calories nor sugar, regulates blood sugar levels,
protects the teeth from decay, strengthens the immune system.
Suitable for diabetics as a sugar substitute.

Grape
Vitamins : C, B1, B2, B6, E, beta-carotene (provitamin A).
Minerals : sodium, potassium, calcium, iron, zinc, magnesium.

Watermelon
Vitamins : A, C.
Minerals : calcium, iron, sodium.

Lemon
Vitamins : C, A, B1, B2, B5, E.
Minerals : calcium, iron, magnesium.

Cinnamon
Can lower blood sugar levels and lower cholesterol levels. At the same time, cinnamon boosts your metabolism, which can be helpful if you want to lose weight. Has a digestive and antibacterial effect and improves blood circulation.

Effect of the ingredients on the organism
VITAMINS

Vitamin A
It strengthens the immune system and good for mucous membranes, eyes, bones, teeth.

Vitamin B1
Good for: metabolism, digestion, heart, memory, wound healing.

Vitamin B2
It strengthens skin and hair, metabolism, eyesight, fertility, thyroid.

Vitamin B5
Provides vitality and energy, strengthens metabolism, hair color pigments, nerves and concentration.

Vitamin B6
Strengthens vitality and immune system, ensures optimal utilization of protein and stable blood sugar.

Vitamin B12
It strengthens the bones, brain and nerves and plays an important role in the formation of muscles and red blood cells. Increases fat burning.

Vitamin C
Fights free radicals (anti-aging effect), strengthens connective tissue, skin, gums and concentration.

Vitamin E
It strengthens the blood circulation and the cardiovascular system, fights free radicals and helps with wound healing and stress management.

Vitamin K
Strengthens the heart function and bone structure, controls blood clotting.

MINERALS

Calcium
It ensures healthy bones and teeth, increases heart function. It contributes to normal muscle function and healthy sleep as well.
It also directs impulses to the nerves.

Iron
It makes an important contribution to the formation of red blood cells and hemoglobin and ensures normal oxygen transport in the body and for a well-functioning immune system. It strengthens the heart function and the immune system.

Potassium
Of central importance for the heart function and muscle contraction, and thus for digestion, muscle activity, the function of the brain and nerves. It ensures the generation of energy, the reduction of pollutants and the maintenance of normal blood pressure.

Copper
It is important for oxygen supply and the formation of antibodies.
It provides the pigmentation of skin and hair. Helps with stress management.

Magnesium
It utilizes carbohydrates and fats for the purpose of energy production and
ensures healthy teeth and bones, normal muscle and nerve function. Besides, it combats tiredness and symptoms of exhaustion.

Manganese
It regulates the metabolism, ensures healthy sleep and good bone structure. Supports the ability to concentrate and

helps in detoxifying the body.

Sodium

Particularly, it is important for nerve conduction and muscle contraction. Regulates the water balance and blood pressure, and influences the activity of certain enzymes.
Phosphorus.
It does not occur in the human body in pure form but in connection with oxygen, in the form of phosphate. Is an important building block of bones and teeth. Has an anti-inflammatory effect and plays a relevant role in the supply of energy.

Zinc

Required for cell division, so it is an important element for skin and connective tissue. Helps with wound healing, strengthens the immune system and the male potency.

THANK YOU

FOR CHOOSING MY RECIPES

AND TRYING OUT

MY DELICIOUS GREEN SMOOTHIES!

CPSIA information can be obtained
at www.ICGtesting.com
Printed in the USA
BVHW091316010621
608554BV00008B/1154